Nurse Report Sh Notebook

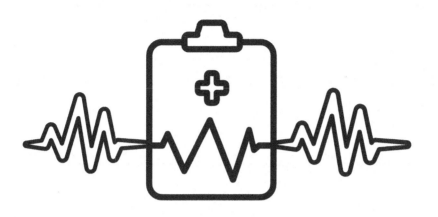

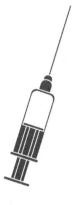

THIS BOOK BELONGS TO:

_____

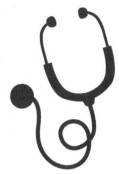

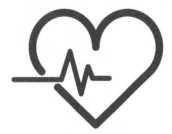

Simply Divine Journals

Nurse Report Sheet

Name:	Code:	Room #:

Allergies:	Isolation:

DX:

PMH:

Neuro:	CV

Resp:	GI/GU:

Skin:	IV'S/Gtt:

Labs:	Notes/Plan:
	• _____
	• _____
	• _____
	• _____
	• _____

Nurse Report Sheet

Name:	Code:	Room #:

Allergies:	Isolation:

DX:

PMH:

Neuro:	CV

Resp:	GI/GU:

Skin:	IV'S/Gtt:

Labs:

Notes/Plan:
- _____
- _____
- _____
- _____
- _____

Nurse Report Sheet

Name:

Code:

Room #:

Allergies:

Isolation:

DX:

PMH:

Neuro:

CV

Resp:

GI/GU:

Skin:

IV'S/Gtt:

Labs:

Notes/Plan:

- _____
- _____
- _____
- _____
- _____

Nurse Report Sheet

Name:

Code:

Room #:

Allergies:

Isolation:

DX:

PMH:

Neuro:

CV

Resp:

GI/GU:

Skin:

IV'S/Gtt:

Labs:

Notes/Plan:
- _____
- _____
- _____
- _____
- _____

Nurse Report Sheet

Name:	Code:	Room #:

Allergies:	Isolation:

DX:

PMH:

Neuro:	CV

Resp:	GI/GU:

Skin:	IV'S/Gtt:

Labs:

Notes/Plan:

- _____
- _____
- _____
- _____
- _____

Nurse Report Sheet

Name:

Code:

Room #:

Allergies:

Isolation:

DX:

PMH:

Neuro:

CV

Resp:

GI/GU:

Skin:

IV'S/Gtt:

Labs:

Notes/Plan:
- _____
- _____
- _____
- _____
- _____

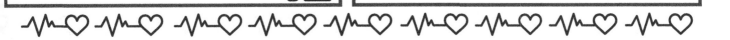

Nurse Report Sheet

Name:

Code:

Room #:

Allergies:

Isolation:

DX:

PMH:

Neuro:

CV

Resp:

GI/GU:

Skin:

IV'S/Gtt:

Labs:

Notes/Plan:
- _____
- _____
- _____
- _____
- _____

Nurse Report Sheet

Name:

Code:

Room #:

Allergies:

Isolation:

DX:

PMH:

Neuro:

CV

Resp:

GI/GU:

Skin:

IV'S/Gtt:

Labs:

Notes/Plan:

- _____
- _____
- _____
- _____
- _____

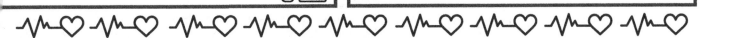

🏥 Nurse Report Sheet 〰️♡

Name:	Code:	Room #:

Allergies:	Isolation:

DX:

PMH:

Neuro:

CV

Resp:

GI/GU:

Skin:

IV'S/Gtt:

Labs:

Notes/Plan:

- _____
- _____
- _____
- _____
- _____

🏥 Nurse Report Sheet 〰️♡

Name:

Code:

Room #:

Allergies:

Isolation:

DX:

PMH:

Neuro:

CV

Resp:

GI/GU:

Skin:

IV'S/Gtt:

Labs:

Notes/Plan:

- _____
- _____
- _____
- _____
- _____

🏥 Nurse Report Sheet ⩘♡

Name:

Code:

Room #:

Allergies:

Isolation:

DX:

PMH:

Neuro:

CV

Resp:

GI/GU:

Skin:

IV'S/Gtt:

Labs:

Notes/Plan:
- _____
- _____
- _____
- _____
- _____

🏥 Nurse Report Sheet 〜♡

Name:	Code:	Room #:

Allergies:	Isolation:

DX:

PMH:

Neuro:	CV

Resp:	GI/GU:

Skin:	IV'S/Gtt:

Labs:	Notes/Plan: • _____ • _____ • _____ • _____ • _____

Nurse Report Sheet

Name:

Code:

Room #:

Allergies:

Isolation:

DX:

PMH:

Neuro:

CV

Resp:

GI/GU:

Skin:

IV'S/Gtt:

Labs:

Notes/Plan:
- _____
- _____
- _____
- _____
- _____

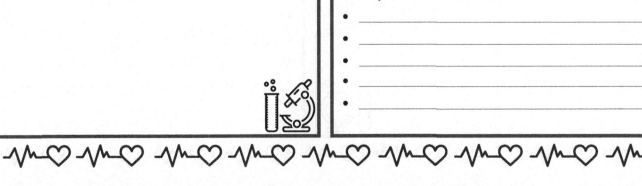

Nurse Report Sheet

Name:

Code:

Room #:

Allergies:

Isolation:

DX:

PMH:

Neuro:

CV

Resp:

GI/GU:

Skin:

IV'S/Gtt:

Labs:

Notes/Plan:

- _____
- _____
- _____
- _____
- _____

Nurse Report Sheet

Name:	Code:	Room #:

Allergies:	Isolation:

DX:

PMH:

Neuro:

CV

Resp:

GI/GU:

Skin:

IV'S/Gtt:

Labs:

Notes/Plan:

- _____
- _____
- _____
- _____
- _____

🪖 Nurse Report Sheet 〜♡

Name:

Code:

Room #:

Allergies:

Isolation:

DX:

PMH:

Neuro:

CV

Resp:

GI/GU:

Skin:

IV'S/Gtt:

Labs:

Notes/Plan:

- _____
- _____
- _____
- _____
- _____

Nurse Report Sheet

Name:	Code:	Room #:

Allergies:	Isolation:

DX:

PMH:

Neuro:	CV

Resp:	GI/GU:

Skin:	IV'S/Gtt:

Labs:	Notes/Plan:

Notes/Plan:
- _____
- _____
- _____
- _____
- _____

Nurse Report Sheet

Name:	Code:	Room #:

Allergies:	Isolation:

DX:

PMH:

Neuro:	CV

Resp:	GI/GU:

Skin:	IV'S/Gtt:

Labs:

Notes/Plan:
- _____
- _____
- _____
- _____
- _____

Nurse Report Sheet

Name:

Code:

Room #:

Allergies:

Isolation:

DX:

PMH:

Neuro:

CV

Resp:

GI/GU:

Skin:

IV'S/Gtt:

Labs:

Notes/Plan:

- _____
- _____
- _____
- _____
- _____

Nurse Report Sheet

Name:

Code:

Room #:

Allergies:

Isolation:

DX:

PMH:

Neuro:

CV

Resp:

GI/GU:

Skin:

IV'S/Gtt:

Labs:

Notes/Plan:

- _____
- _____
- _____
- _____
- _____

Nurse Report Sheet

Name:

Code:

Room #:

Allergies:

Isolation:

DX:

PMH:

Neuro:

CV

Resp:

GI/GU:

Skin:

IV'S/Gtt:

Labs:

Notes/Plan:
- _____
- _____
- _____
- _____
- _____

Nurse Report Sheet

Name:

Code:

Room #:

Allergies:

Isolation:

DX:

PMH:

Neuro:

CV

Resp:

GI/GU:

Skin:

IV'S/Gtt:

Labs:

Notes/Plan:

- _____
- _____
- _____
- _____
- _____

🧑‍⚕️ Nurse Report Sheet 〰️♡

Name:

Code:

Room #:

Allergies:

Isolation:

DX:

PMH:

Neuro:

CV

Resp:

GI/GU:

Skin:

IV'S/Gtt:

Labs:

Notes/Plan:

- _____
- _____
- _____
- _____
- _____

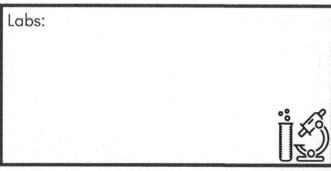

Nurse Report Sheet

Name:

Code:

Room #:

Allergies:

Isolation:

DX:

PMH:

Neuro:

CV

Resp:

GI/GU:

Skin:

IV'S/Gtt:

Labs:

Notes/Plan:

- _____
- _____
- _____
- _____
- _____

Nurse Report Sheet

Name:	Code:	Room #:

Allergies:	Isolation:

DX:

PMH:

Neuro:	CV

Resp:	GI/GU:

Skin:	IV'S/Gtt:

Labs:

Notes/Plan:
- _____
- _____
- _____
- _____
- _____

Nurse Report Sheet

Name:

Code:

Room #:

Allergies:

Isolation:

DX:

PMH:

Neuro:

CV

Resp:

GI/GU:

Skin:

IV'S/Gtt:

Labs:

Notes/Plan:

- _____
- _____
- _____
- _____
- _____

🎩 Nurse Report Sheet ⚕️♡

Name:

Code:

Room #:

Allergies:

Isolation:

DX:

PMH:

Neuro:

CV

Resp:

GI/GU:

Skin:

IV'S/Gtt:

Labs:

Notes/Plan:

- _____
- _____
- _____
- _____
- _____

Nurse Report Sheet

Name:

Code:

Room #:

Allergies:

Isolation:

DX:

PMH:

Neuro:

CV

Resp:

GI/GU:

Skin:

IV'S/Gtt:

Labs:

Notes/Plan:

- _____
- _____
- _____
- _____
- _____

🏥 Nurse Report Sheet ⎍♡

Name: _____ | **Code:** _____ | **Room #:** _____

Allergies: _____ | **Isolation:** _____

DX:

PMH:

Neuro:	CV

Resp:	GI/GU:

Skin:	IV'S/Gtt:

Labs:	Notes/Plan:

Notes/Plan:
- _____
- _____
- _____
- _____
- _____

Nurse Report Sheet

Name:

Code:

Room #:

Allergies:

Isolation:

DX:

PMH:

Neuro:

CV

Resp:

GI/GU:

Skin:

IV'S/Gtt:

Labs:

Notes/Plan:

- _____
- _____
- _____
- _____
- _____

🩺 Nurse Report Sheet ⎍♡

Name: Code: Room #:

Allergies: Isolation:

DX:

PMH:

Neuro: CV

Resp: GI/GU:

Skin: IV'S/Gtt:

Labs: Notes/Plan:
                                 • _____
                                 • _____
                                 • _____
                                 • _____
                                 • _____

Nurse Report Sheet

Name:

Code:

Room #:

Allergies:

Isolation:

DX:

PMH:

Neuro:

CV

Resp:

GI/GU:

Skin:

IV'S/Gtt:

Labs:

Notes/Plan:

- _____
- _____
- _____
- _____
- _____

🎩 Nurse Report Sheet ⚡♡

Name:

Code:

Room #:

Allergies:

Isolation:

DX:

PMH:

Neuro:

CV

Resp:

GI/GU:

Skin:

IV'S/Gtt:

Labs:

Notes/Plan:

- _____
- _____
- _____
- _____
- _____

Nurse Report Sheet

Name:

Code:

Room #:

Allergies:

Isolation:

DX:

PMH:

Neuro:

CV

Resp:

GI/GU:

Skin:

IV'S/Gtt:

Labs:

Notes/Plan:

- _____
- _____
- _____
- _____
- _____

🩺 Nurse Report Sheet ⌁♡

Name: | **Code:** | **Room #:**

Allergies: | **Isolation:**

DX:

PMH:

Neuro: | **CV**

Resp: | **GI/GU:**

Skin: | **IV'S/Gtt:**

Labs: | **Notes/Plan:**
- _____
- _____
- _____
- _____
- _____

Nurse Report Sheet

Name:

Code:

Room #:

Allergies:

Isolation:

DX:

PMH:

Neuro:

CV

Resp:

GI/GU:

Skin:

IV'S/Gtt:

Labs:

Notes/Plan:

- _____
- _____
- _____
- _____
- _____

🩺 Nurse Report Sheet ⩘♡

Name:	Code:	Room #:

Allergies:

Isolation:

DX:

PMH:

Neuro:

CV

Resp:

GI/GU:

Skin:

IV'S/Gtt:

Labs:

Notes/Plan:
- _____
- _____
- _____
- _____
- _____

Nurse Report Sheet

Name:	Code:	Room #:

Allergies:	Isolation:

DX:

PMH:

Neuro:	CV

Resp:	GI/GU:

Skin:	IV'S/Gtt:

Labs:	Notes/Plan:
	• _____
	• _____
	• _____
	• _____
	• _____

Nurse Report Sheet

Name:

Code:

Room #:

Allergies:

Isolation:

DX:

PMH:

Neuro:

CV

Resp:

GI/GU:

Skin:

IV'S/Gtt:

Labs:

Notes/Plan:

- _____
- _____
- _____
- _____
- _____

Nurse Report Sheet

Name:

Code:

Room #:

Allergies:

Isolation:

DX:

PMH:

Neuro:

CV

Resp:

GI/GU:

Skin:

IV'S/Gtt:

Labs:

Notes/Plan:

- _____
- _____
- _____
- _____
- _____

Nurse Report Sheet

Name:	Code:	Room #:

Allergies:	Isolation:

DX:

PMH:

Neuro:	CV

Resp:	GI/GU:

Skin:	IV'S/Gtt:

Labs:

Notes/Plan:
- _____
- _____
- _____
- _____
- _____

Nurse Report Sheet

Name:

Code:

Room #:

Allergies:

Isolation:

DX:

PMH:

Neuro:

CV

Resp:

GI/GU:

Skin:

IV'S/Gtt:

Labs:

Notes/Plan:

- _____
- _____
- _____
- _____
- _____

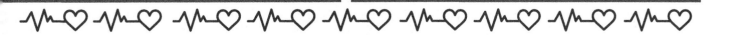

Nurse Report Sheet

Name:	Code:	Room #:

Allergies:	Isolation:

DX:

PMH:

Neuro:	CV

Resp:	GI/GU:

Skin:	IV'S/Gtt:

Labs:

Notes/Plan:
- _____
- _____
- _____
- _____
- _____

Nurse Report Sheet

| Name: | Code: | Room #: |

| Allergies: | Isolation: |

DX:

PMH:

| Neuro: | CV |

| Resp: | GI/GU: |

| Skin: | IV'S/Gtt: |

Labs:

Notes/Plan:

- _____
- _____
- _____
- _____
- _____

🏥 Nurse Report Sheet ⩘♡

Name:

Code:

Room #:

Allergies:

Isolation:

DX:

PMH:

Neuro:

CV

Resp:

GI/GU:

Skin:

IV'S/Gtt:

Labs:

Notes/Plan:
- _____
- _____
- _____
- _____
- _____

Nurse Report Sheet

Name:

Code:

Room #:

Allergies:

Isolation:

DX:

PMH:

Neuro:

CV

Resp:

GI/GU:

Skin:

IV'S/Gtt:

Labs:

Notes/Plan:

- _____
- _____
- _____
- _____
- _____

Nurse Report Sheet

Name:

Code:

Room #:

Allergies:

Isolation:

DX:

PMH:

Neuro:

CV

Resp:

GI/GU:

Skin:

IV'S/Gtt:

Labs:

Notes/Plan:
- _____
- _____
- _____
- _____
- _____

Nurse Report Sheet

Name:	Code:	Room #:

Allergies:	Isolation:

DX:

PMH:

Neuro:	CV

Resp:	GI/GU:

Skin:	IV'S/Gtt:

Labs:	Notes/Plan:

Notes/Plan:
- _____
- _____
- _____
- _____
- _____

Nurse Report Sheet

Name:	Code:	Room #:

Allergies:	Isolation:

DX:

PMH:

Neuro:	CV

Resp:	GI/GU:

Skin:	IV'S/Gtt:

Labs:

Notes/Plan:
- _____
- _____
- _____
- _____
- _____

Nurse Report Sheet

Name:

Code:

Room #:

Allergies:

Isolation:

DX:

PMH:

Neuro:

CV

Resp:

GI/GU:

Skin:

IV'S/Gtt:

Labs:

Notes/Plan:

- _____
- _____
- _____
- _____
- _____

Nurse Report Sheet

Name:	Code:	Room #:

Allergies:	Isolation:

DX:

PMH:

Neuro:	CV

Resp:	GI/GU:

Skin:	IV'S/Gtt:

Labs:	Notes/Plan:

Notes/Plan:
- _____
- _____
- _____
- _____
- _____

Nurse Report Sheet

| Name: | Code: | Room #: |

Allergies: | **Isolation:**

DX:

PMH:

Neuro: | **CV**

Resp: | **GI/GU:**

Skin: | **IV'S/Gtt:**

Labs: | **Notes/Plan:**
- _____
- _____
- _____
- _____
- _____

🩺 Nurse Report Sheet 〰️♡

Name:

Code:

Room #:

Allergies:

Isolation:

DX:

PMH:

Neuro:

CV

Resp:

GI/GU:

Skin:

IV'S/Gtt:

Labs:

Notes/Plan:

- _____
- _____
- _____
- _____
- _____

Nurse Report Sheet

Name:	Code:	Room #:

Allergies:	Isolation:

DX:

PMH:

Neuro:

CV

Resp:

GI/GU:

Skin:

IV'S/Gtt:

Labs:

Notes/Plan:
- _____
- _____
- _____
- _____
- _____

Nurse Report Sheet

Name:

Code:

Room #:

Allergies:

Isolation:

DX:

PMH:

Neuro:

CV

Resp:

GI/GU:

Skin:

IV'S/Gtt:

Labs:

Notes/Plan:

- _____
- _____
- _____
- _____
- _____

Nurse Report Sheet

Name:	Code:	Room #:

Allergies:	Isolation:

DX:

PMH:

Neuro:	CV

Resp:	GI/GU:

Skin:	IV'S/Gtt:

Labs:

Notes/Plan:
- _____
- _____
- _____
- _____
- _____

Nurse Report Sheet

Name:

Code:

Room #:

Allergies:

Isolation:

DX:

PMH:

Neuro:

CV

Resp:

GI/GU:

Skin:

IV'S/Gtt:

Labs:

Notes/Plan:
- _____
- _____
- _____
- _____
- _____

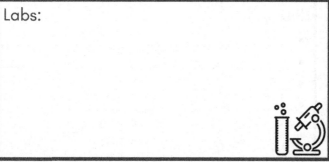

Nurse Report Sheet

Name:	Code:	Room #:

Allergies:	Isolation:

DX:

PMH:

Neuro:

CV

Resp:

GI/GU:

Skin:

IV'S/Gtt:

Labs:

Notes/Plan:

- _____
- _____
- _____
- _____
- _____

🏥 Nurse Report Sheet 〰️♡

Name:

Code:

Room #:

Allergies:

Isolation:

DX:

PMH:

Neuro:

CV

Resp:

GI/GU:

Skin:

IV'S/Gtt:

Labs:

Notes/Plan:

- _____
- _____
- _____
- _____
- _____

Nurse Report Sheet

Name:

Code:

Room #:

Allergies:

Isolation:

DX:

PMH:

Neuro:

CV

Resp:

GI/GU:

Skin:

IV'S/Gtt:

Labs:

Notes/Plan:

- _____
- _____
- _____
- _____
- _____

Nurse Report Sheet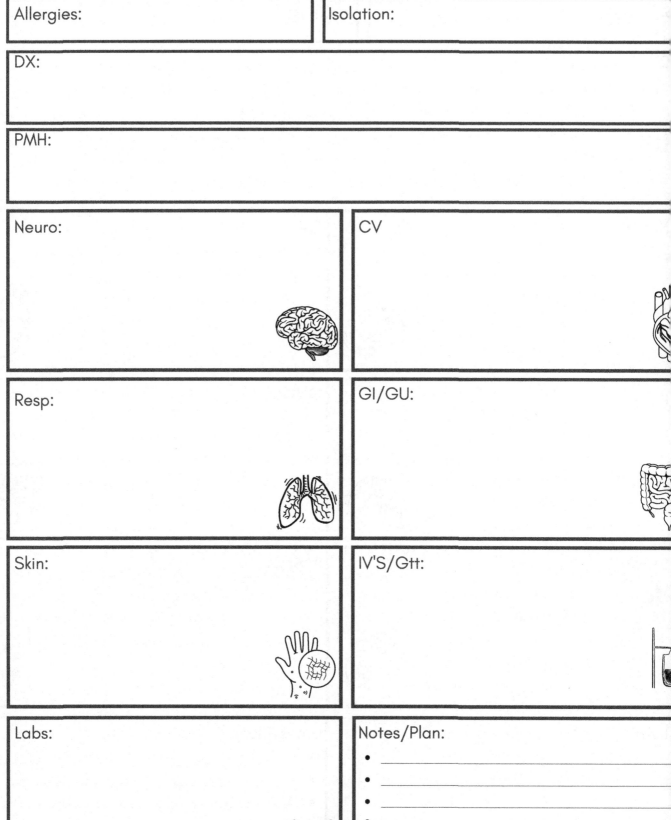

Name:

Code:

Room #:

Allergies:

Isolation:

DX:

PMH:

Neuro:

CV

Resp:

GI/GU:

Skin:

IV'S/Gtt:

Labs:

Notes/Plan:
- _____
- _____
- _____
- _____
- _____

Nurse Report Sheet

Name:

Code:

Room #:

Allergies:

Isolation:

DX:

PMH:

Neuro:

CV

Resp:

GI/GU:

Skin:

IV'S/Gtt:

Labs:

Notes/Plan:

- _____
- _____
- _____
- _____
- _____

Nurse Report Sheet

Name:

Code:

Room #:

Allergies:

Isolation:

DX:

PMH:

Neuro:

CV

Resp:

GI/GU:

Skin:

IV'S/Gtt:

Labs:

Notes/Plan:
- _____
- _____
- _____
- _____
- _____

Nurse Report Sheet

Name:	Code:	Room #:

Allergies:	Isolation:

DX:

PMH:

Neuro:

CV

Resp:

GI/GU:

Skin:

IV'S/Gtt:

Labs:

Notes/Plan:
- _____
- _____
- _____
- _____
- _____

Nurse Report Sheet

Name:	Code:	Room #:

Allergies:	Isolation:

DX:

PMH:

Neuro:

CV

Resp:

GI/GU:

Skin:

IV'S/Gtt:

Labs:

Notes/Plan:
- _____
- _____
- _____
- _____
- _____

Nurse Report Sheet

Name:	Code:	Room #:

Allergies:	Isolation:

DX:

PMH:

Neuro:	CV

Resp:	GI/GU:

Skin:	IV'S/Gtt:

Labs:

Notes/Plan:
- _____
- _____
- _____
- _____
- _____

🏥 Nurse Report Sheet 〰♡

| Name: | Code: | Room #: |

| Allergies: | Isolation: |

DX:

PMH:

Neuro:

CV

Resp:

GI/GU:

Skin:

IV'S/Gtt:

Labs:

Notes/Plan:
- _____
- _____
- _____
- _____
- _____

🧢 Nurse Report Sheet ⩓♡

Name:

Code:

Room #:

Allergies:

Isolation:

DX:

PMH:

Neuro:

CV

Resp:

GI/GU:

Skin:

IV'S/Gtt:

Labs:

Notes/Plan:

- _____
- _____
- _____
- _____
- _____

🏥 Nurse Report Sheet 〰️♡

Name:

Code:

Room #:

Allergies:

Isolation:

DX:

PMH:

Neuro:

CV

Resp:

GI/GU:

Skin:

IV'S/Gtt:

Labs:

Notes/Plan:

- _____
- _____
- _____
- _____
- _____

Nurse Report Sheet

Name:

Code:

Room #:

Allergies:

Isolation:

DX:

PMH:

Neuro:

CV

Resp:

GI/GU:

Skin:

IV'S/Gtt:

Labs:

Notes/Plan:

- _____
- _____
- _____
- _____
- _____

Nurse Report Sheet

Name:

Code:

Room #:

Allergies:

Isolation:

DX:

PMH:

Neuro:

CV

Resp:

GI/GU:

Skin:

IV'S/Gtt:

Labs:

Notes/Plan:
- _____
- _____
- _____
- _____
- _____

🧑‍⚕️ Nurse Report Sheet ⏜♡

Name:

Code:

Room #:

Allergies:

Isolation:

DX:

PMH:

Neuro:

CV

Resp:

GI/GU:

Skin:

IV'S/Gtt:

Labs:

Notes/Plan:

- _____
- _____
- _____
- _____
- _____

Nurse Report Sheet

Name:

Code:

Room #:

Allergies:

Isolation:

DX:

PMH:

Neuro:

CV

Resp:

GI/GU:

Skin:

IV'S/Gtt:

Labs:

Notes/Plan:

- _____
- _____
- _____
- _____
- _____

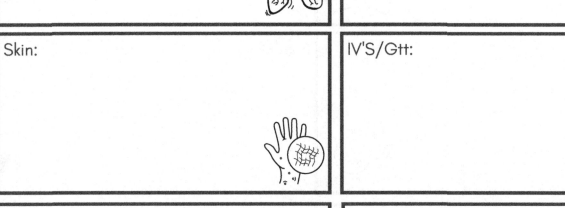
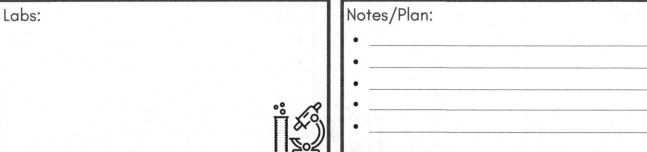

🏥 Nurse Report Sheet ⎓♡

Name:

Code:

Room #:

Allergies:

Isolation:

DX:

PMH:

Neuro:

CV

Resp:

GI/GU:

Skin:

IV'S/Gtt:

Labs:

Notes/Plan:
- _____
- _____
- _____
- _____
- _____

🩺 Nurse Report Sheet ⎯╲╱⎯♡

Name:

Code:

Room #:

Allergies:

Isolation:

DX:

PMH:

Neuro:

CV

Resp:

GI/GU:

Skin:

IV'S/Gtt:

Labs:

Notes/Plan:
- _____
- _____
- _____
- _____
- _____

🧢 Nurse Report Sheet ⚕️♡

Name:

Code:

Room #:

Allergies:

Isolation:

DX:

PMH:

Neuro:

CV

Resp:

GI/GU:

Skin:

IV'S/Gtt:

Labs:

Notes/Plan:

- _____
- _____
- _____
- _____
- _____

Nurse Report Sheet

Name:	Code:	Room #:

Allergies:	Isolation:

DX:

PMH:

Neuro:	CV

Resp:	GI/GU:

Skin:	IV'S/Gtt:

Labs:	Notes/Plan:

Notes/Plan:
- _____
- _____
- _____
- _____
- _____

🪖 Nurse Report Sheet 〰️♡

Name: | **Code:** | **Room #:**

Allergies: | **Isolation:**

DX:

PMH:

Neuro: | **CV**

Resp: | **GI/GU:**

Skin: | **IV'S/Gtt:**

Labs: | **Notes/Plan:**
- _____
- _____
- _____
- _____
- _____

Nurse Report Sheet

Name:

Code:

Room #:

Allergies:

Isolation:

DX:

PMH:

Neuro:

CV

Resp:

GI/GU:

Skin:

IV'S/Gtt:

Labs:

Notes/Plan:
- _____
- _____
- _____
- _____
- _____

Nurse Report Sheet

Name:

Code:

Room #:

Allergies:

Isolation:

DX:

PMH:

Neuro:

CV

Resp:

GI/GU:

Skin:

IV'S/Gtt:

Labs:

Notes/Plan:

- _____
- _____
- _____
- _____
- _____

Nurse Report Sheet

Name:	Code:	Room #:

Allergies:	Isolation:

DX:

PMH:

Neuro:	CV

Resp:	GI/GU:

Skin:	IV'S/Gtt:

Labs:

Notes/Plan:
- _____
- _____
- _____
- _____
- _____

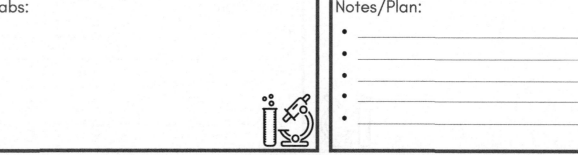

Nurse Report Sheet

Name:

Code:

Room #:

Allergies:

Isolation:

DX:

PMH:

Neuro:

CV

Resp:

GI/GU:

Skin:

IV'S/Gtt:

Labs:

Notes/Plan:

- _____
- _____
- _____
- _____
- _____

Nurse Report Sheet

Name:	Code:	Room #:

Allergies:	Isolation:

DX:

PMH:

Neuro:

CV

Resp:

GI/GU:

Skin:

IV'S/Gtt:

Labs:

Notes/Plan:

- _____
- _____
- _____
- _____
- _____

Nurse Report Sheet

Name:

Code:

Room #:

Allergies:

Isolation:

DX:

PMH:

Neuro:

CV

Resp:

GI/GU:

Skin:

IV'S/Gtt:

Labs:

Notes/Plan:

- _____
- _____
- _____
- _____
- _____

🏥 Nurse Report Sheet ⩓♡

Name:

Code:

Room #:

Allergies:

Isolation:

DX:

PMH:

Neuro:

CV

Resp:

GI/GU:

Skin:

IV'S/Gtt:

Labs:

Notes/Plan:
- _____
- _____
- _____
- _____
- _____

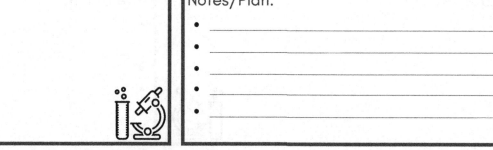

Nurse Report Sheet

Name:

Code:

Room #:

Allergies:

Isolation:

DX:

PMH:

Neuro:

CV

Resp:

GI/GU:

Skin:

IV'S/Gtt:

Labs:

Notes/Plan:

- _____
- _____
- _____
- _____
- _____

Nurse Report Sheet

Name:	Code:	Room #:

Allergies:	Isolation:

DX:

PMH:

Neuro:	CV

Resp:	GI/GU:

Skin:	IV'S/Gtt:

Labs:

Notes/Plan:
- _____
- _____
- _____
- _____
- _____

Nurse Report Sheet

Name:

Code:

Room #:

Allergies:

Isolation:

DX:

PMH:

Neuro:

CV

Resp:

GI/GU:

Skin:

IV'S/Gtt:

Labs:

Notes/Plan:

- _____
- _____
- _____
- _____
- _____

Nurse Report Sheet

Name:	Code:	Room #:

Allergies:	Isolation:

DX:

PMH:

Neuro:	CV

Resp:	GI/GU:

Skin:	IV'S/Gtt:

Labs:	Notes/Plan:

Notes/Plan:
- _____
- _____
- _____
- _____
- _____

Nurse Report Sheet

| Name: | Code: | Room #: |

Allergies:

Isolation:

DX:

PMH:

Neuro:

CV

Resp:

GI/GU:

Skin:

IV'S/Gtt:

Labs:

Notes/Plan:
- _____
- _____
- _____
- _____
- _____

Nurse Report Sheet

Name:

Code:

Room #:

Allergies:

Isolation:

DX:

PMH:

Neuro:

CV

Resp:

GI/GU:

Skin:

IV'S/Gtt:

Labs:

Notes/Plan:
- _____
- _____
- _____
- _____
- _____

Nurse Report Sheet

Name:	Code:	Room #:

Allergies:	Isolation:

DX:

PMH:

Neuro:	CV

Resp:	GI/GU:

Skin:	IV'S/Gtt:

Labs:	Notes/Plan:

Notes/Plan:
- _____
- _____
- _____
- _____
- _____

Nurse Report Sheet

Name:	Code:	Room #:

Allergies:	Isolation:

DX:

PMH:

Neuro:

CV

Resp:

GI/GU:

Skin:

IV'S/Gtt:

Labs:

Notes/Plan:
- _____
- _____
- _____
- _____
- _____

Nurse Report Sheet

Name:

Code:

Room #:

Allergies:

Isolation:

DX:

PMH:

Neuro:

CV

Resp:

GI/GU:

Skin:

IV'S/Gtt:

Labs:

Notes/Plan:
- _____
- _____
- _____
- _____
- _____

🏥 Nurse Report Sheet 〜♡

Name:

Code:

Room #:

Allergies:

Isolation:

DX:

PMH:

Neuro:

CV

Resp:

GI/GU:

Skin:

IV'S/Gtt:

Labs:

Notes/Plan:
- _____
- _____
- _____
- _____
- _____

Nurse Report Sheet

Name:

Code:

Room #:

Allergies:

Isolation:

DX:

PMH:

Neuro:

CV

Resp:

GI/GU:

Skin:

IV'S/Gtt:

Labs:

Notes/Plan:

- _____
- _____
- _____
- _____
- _____

Nurse Report Sheet

Name:

Code:

Room #:

Allergies:

Isolation:

DX:

PMH:

Neuro:

CV

Resp:

GI/GU:

Skin:

IV'S/Gtt:

Labs:

Notes/Plan:
- _____
- _____
- _____
- _____
- _____

Nurse Report Sheet

Name:

Code:

Room #:

Allergies:

Isolation:

DX:

PMH:

Neuro:

CV

Resp:

GI/GU:

Skin:

IV'S/Gtt:

Labs:

Notes/Plan:
- _____
- _____
- _____
- _____
- _____

Nurse Report Sheet

Name:	Code:	Room #:

Allergies:	Isolation:

DX:

PMH:

Neuro:	CV

Resp:	GI/GU:

Skin:	IV'S/Gtt:

Labs:

Notes/Plan:
- _____
- _____
- _____
- _____
- _____

🩺 Nurse Report Sheet 〰️♡

Name:

Code:

Room #:

Allergies:

Isolation:

DX:

PMH:

Neuro:

CV

Resp:

GI/GU:

Skin:

IV'S/Gtt:

Labs:

Notes/Plan:

- _____
- _____
- _____
- _____
- _____

Nurse Report Sheet

Name:

Code:

Room #:

Allergies:

Isolation:

DX:

PMH:

Neuro:

CV

Resp:

GI/GU:

Skin:

IV'S/Gtt:

Labs:

Notes/Plan:
- _____
- _____
- _____
- _____
- _____

Nurse Report Sheet

Name:	Code:	Room #:

Allergies:	Isolation:

DX:

PMH:

Neuro:	CV

Resp:	GI/GU:

Skin:	IV'S/Gtt:

Labs:	Notes/Plan:

Notes/Plan:
- _____
- _____
- _____
- _____
- _____

Nurse Report Sheet

Name:	Code:	Room #:

Allergies:	Isolation:

DX:

PMH:

Neuro:

CV

Resp:

GI/GU:

Skin:

IV'S/Gtt:

Labs:

Notes/Plan:
- _____
- _____
- _____
- _____
- _____

Nurse Report Sheet

Name:

Code:

Room #:

Allergies:

Isolation:

DX:

PMH:

Neuro:

CV

Resp:

GI/GU:

Skin:

IV'S/Gtt:

Labs:

Notes/Plan:

- _____
- _____
- _____
- _____
- _____

Nurse Report Sheet

Name:

Code:

Room #:

Allergies:

Isolation:

DX:

PMH:

Neuro:

CV

Resp:

GI/GU:

Skin:

IV'S/Gtt:

Labs:

Notes/Plan:
- _____
- _____
- _____
- _____
- _____

Nurse Report Sheet

Name:

Code:

Room #:

Allergies:

Isolation:

DX:

PMH:

Neuro:

CV

Resp:

GI/GU:

Skin:

IV'S/Gtt:

Labs:

Notes/Plan:
- _____
- _____
- _____
- _____
- _____

🩺 Nurse Report Sheet 〰️♡

Name:

Code:

Room #:

Allergies:

Isolation:

DX:

PMH:

Neuro:

CV

Resp:

GI/GU:

Skin:

IV'S/Gtt:

Labs:

Notes/Plan:
- _____
- _____
- _____
- _____
- _____

Nurse Report Sheet

Name:	Code:	Room #:

Allergies:	Isolation:

DX:

PMH:

Neuro:	CV

Resp:	GI/GU:

Skin:	IV'S/Gtt:

Labs:	Notes/Plan:

Notes/Plan:
- _____
- _____
- _____
- _____
- _____

Nurse Report Sheet

Name:

Code:

Room #:

Allergies:

Isolation:

DX:

PMH:

Neuro:

CV

Resp:

GI/GU:

Skin:

IV'S/Gtt:

Labs:

Notes/Plan:

- _____
- _____
- _____
- _____
- _____

Nurse Report Sheet

Name:

Code:

Room #:

Allergies:

Isolation:

DX:

PMH:

Neuro:

CV

Resp:

GI/GU:

Skin:

IV'S/Gtt:

Labs:

Notes/Plan:

- _____
- _____
- _____
- _____
- _____

Nurse Report Sheet

Name:	Code:	Room #:

Allergies:	Isolation:

DX:

PMH:

Neuro:	CV

Resp:	GI/GU:

Skin:	IV'S/Gtt:

Labs:

Notes/Plan:
- _____
- _____
- _____
- _____
- _____

Nurse Report Sheet

Name:	Code:	Room #:

Allergies:	Isolation:

DX:

PMH:

Neuro:	CV

Resp:	GI/GU:

Skin:	IV'S/Gtt:

Labs:	Notes/Plan:
	• _____
	• _____
	• _____
	• _____
	• _____

Nurse Report Sheet

Name:	Code:	Room #:

Allergies:	Isolation:

DX:

PMH:

Neuro:	CV

Resp:	GI/GU:

Skin:	IV'S/Gtt:

Labs:

Notes/Plan:
- _____
- _____
- _____
- _____
- _____

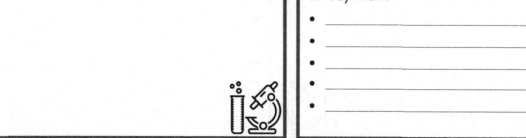

Nurse Report Sheet

Name:

Code:

Room #:

Allergies:

Isolation:

DX:

PMH:

Neuro:

CV

Resp:

GI/GU:

Skin:

IV'S/Gtt:

Labs:

Notes/Plan:
- _____
- _____
- _____
- _____
- _____

Nurse Report Sheet

Name:

Code:

Room #:

Allergies:

Isolation:

DX:

PMH:

Neuro:

CV

Resp:

GI/GU:

Skin:

IV'S/Gtt:

Labs:

Notes/Plan:
- _____
- _____
- _____
- _____
- _____

Nurse Report Sheet

Name:	Code:	Room #:

Allergies:	Isolation:

DX:

PMH:

Neuro:	CV

Resp:	GI/GU:

Skin:	IV'S/Gtt:

Labs:	Notes/Plan:

Notes/Plan:
- _____
- _____
- _____
- _____
- _____

Nurse Report Sheet

Name:

Code:

Room #:

Allergies:

Isolation:

DX:

PMH:

Neuro:

CV

Resp:

GI/GU:

Skin:

IV'S/Gtt:

Labs:

Notes/Plan:

- _____
- _____
- _____
- _____
- _____

Nurse Report Sheet

Name:

Code:

Room #:

Allergies:

Isolation:

DX:

PMH:

Neuro:

CV

Resp:

GI/GU:

Skin:

IV'S/Gtt:

Labs:

Notes/Plan:

- _____
- _____
- _____
- _____
- _____

🏥 Nurse Report Sheet ⚡♡

Name: | Code: | Room #:

Allergies: | Isolation:

DX:

PMH:

Neuro: | CV

Resp: | GI/GU:

Skin: | IV'S/Gtt:

Labs: | Notes/Plan:
- _____
- _____
- _____
- _____
- _____

🩺 Nurse Report Sheet ⎓♡

Name:

Code:

Room #:

Allergies:

Isolation:

DX:

PMH:

Neuro:

CV

Resp:

GI/GU:

Skin:

IV'S/Gtt:

Labs:

Notes/Plan:

- _____
- _____
- _____
- _____
- _____

⚕ Nurse Report Sheet ∿♡

Name:

Code:

Room #:

Allergies:

Isolation:

DX:

PMH:

Neuro:

CV

Resp:

GI/GU:

Skin:

IV'S/Gtt:

Labs:

Notes/Plan:

- _____
- _____
- _____
- _____
- _____

Nurse Report Sheet

Name:	Code:	Room #:

Allergies:	Isolation:

DX:

PMH:

Neuro:	CV

Resp:	GI/GU:

Skin:	IV'S/Gtt:

Labs:

Notes/Plan:
- _____
- _____
- _____
- _____
- _____

Nurse Report Sheet

Name:	Code:	Room #:

Allergies:	Isolation:

DX:

PMH:

Neuro:	CV

Resp:	GI/GU:

Skin:	IV'S/Gtt:

Labs:	Notes/Plan:

Notes/Plan:
- _____
- _____
- _____
- _____
- _____

🩺 Nurse Report Sheet 〰♡

Name:

Code:

Room #:

Allergies:

Isolation:

DX:

PMH:

Neuro:

CV

Resp:

GI/GU:

Skin:

IV'S/Gtt:

Labs:

Notes/Plan:

- _____
- _____
- _____
- _____
- _____

🏥 Nurse Report Sheet ⩘♡

Name: Code: Room #:

Allergies: Isolation:

DX:

PMH:

Neuro: CV

Resp: GI/GU:

Skin: IV'S/Gtt:

Labs: Notes/Plan:
                                 • _____
                                 • _____
                                 • _____
                                 • _____
                                 • _____

Nurse Report Sheet

Name:	Code:	Room #:

Allergies:	Isolation:

DX:

PMH:

Neuro:	CV

Resp:	GI/GU:

Skin:	IV'S/Gtt:

Labs:	Notes/Plan:
	• _____
	• _____
	• _____
	• _____
	• _____

Nurse Report Sheet

Name:

Code:

Room #:

Allergies:

Isolation:

DX:

PMH:

Neuro:

CV

Resp:

GI/GU:

Skin:

IV'S/Gtt:

Labs:

Notes/Plan:

- _____
- _____
- _____
- _____
- _____

Nurse Report Sheet

Name:

Code:

Room #:

Allergies:

Isolation:

DX:

PMH:

Neuro:

CV

Resp:

GI/GU:

Skin:

IV'S/Gtt:

Labs:

Notes/Plan:

- _____
- _____
- _____
- _____
- _____

Nurse Report Sheet

Name:

Code:

Room #:

Allergies:

Isolation:

DX:

PMH:

Neuro:

CV

Resp:

GI/GU:

Skin:

IV'S/Gtt:

Labs:

Notes/Plan:
- _____
- _____
- _____
- _____
- _____

Nurse Report Sheet

Name:

Code:

Room #:

Allergies:

Isolation:

DX:

PMH:

Neuro:

CV

Resp:

GI/GU:

Skin:

IV'S/Gtt:

Labs:

Notes/Plan:

- _____
- _____
- _____
- _____
- _____

Nurse Report Sheet

Name:

Code:

Room #:

Allergies:

Isolation:

DX:

PMH:

Neuro:

CV

Resp:

GI/GU:

Skin:

IV'S/Gtt:

Labs:

Notes/Plan:

- _____
- _____
- _____
- _____
- _____

Nurse Report Sheet

Name:

Code:

Room #:

Allergies:

Isolation:

DX:

PMH:

Neuro:

CV

Resp:

GI/GU:

Skin:

IV'S/Gtt:

Labs:

Notes/Plan:

- _____
- _____
- _____
- _____
- _____

🏥 Nurse Report Sheet 〰♡

Name: _____ Code: _____ Room #: _____

Allergies: _____ Isolation: _____

DX:

PMH:

Neuro:	CV
Resp:	GI/GU:
Skin:	IV'S/Gtt:
Labs:	Notes/Plan: • _____ • _____ • _____ • _____ • _____

Nurse Report Sheet

Name:

Code:

Room #:

Allergies:

Isolation:

DX:

PMH:

Neuro:

CV

Resp:

GI/GU:

Skin:

IV'S/Gtt:

Labs:

Notes/Plan:

- _____
- _____
- _____
- _____
- _____

Nurse Report Sheet

Name:	Code:	Room #:

Allergies:	Isolation:

DX:

PMH:

Neuro:	CV

Resp:	GI/GU:

Skin:	IV'S/Gtt:

Labs:

Notes/Plan:
- _____
- _____
- _____
- _____
- _____

Nurse Report Sheet

Name:	Code:	Room #:

Allergies:	Isolation:

DX:

PMH:

Neuro:	CV

Resp:	GI/GU:

Skin:	IV'S/Gtt:

Labs:	Notes/Plan:

Notes/Plan:
- _____
- _____
- _____
- _____
- _____

Nurse Report Sheet

Name:

Code:

Room #:

Allergies:

Isolation:

DX:

PMH:

Neuro:

CV

Resp:

GI/GU:

Skin:

IV'S/Gtt:

Labs:

Notes/Plan:

- _____
- _____
- _____
- _____
- _____

☤ Nurse Report Sheet ⎍♡

Name:	Code:	Room #:

Allergies:	Isolation:

DX:

PMH:

Neuro:	CV

Resp:	GI/GU:

Skin:	IV'S/Gtt:

Labs:

Notes/Plan:
- _____
- _____
- _____
- _____
- _____

Nurse Report Sheet

Name:	Code:	Room #:

Allergies:	Isolation:

DX:

PMH:

Neuro:	CV

Resp:	GI/GU:

Skin:	IV'S/Gtt:

Labs:	Notes/Plan:

Notes/Plan:
- _____
- _____
- _____
- _____
- _____

Nurse Report Sheet

Name:

Code:

Room #:

Allergies:

Isolation:

DX:

PMH:

Neuro:

CV

Resp:

GI/GU:

Skin:

IV'S/Gtt:

Labs:

Notes/Plan:

- _____
- _____
- _____
- _____
- _____

🩺 Nurse Report Sheet ⚡♡

Name:

Code:

Room #:

Allergies:

Isolation:

DX:

PMH:

Neuro:

CV

Resp:

GI/GU:

Skin:

IV'S/Gtt:

Labs:

Notes/Plan:

- _____
- _____
- _____
- _____
- _____

Nurse Report Sheet

Name:	Code:	Room #:

Allergies:	Isolation:

DX:

PMH:

Neuro:	CV

Resp:	GI/GU:

Skin:	IV'S/Gtt:

Labs:

Notes/Plan:

- _____
- _____
- _____
- _____
- _____

Nurse Report Sheet

Name:	Code:	Room #:

Allergies:	Isolation:

DX:

PMH:

Neuro:	CV

Resp:	GI/GU:

Skin:	IV'S/Gtt:

Labs:	Notes/Plan:

Notes/Plan:
- _____
- _____
- _____
- _____
- _____

Nurse Report Sheet

Name:

Code:

Room #:

Allergies:

Isolation:

DX:

PMH:

Neuro:

CV

Resp:

GI/GU:

Skin:

IV'S/Gtt:

Labs:

Notes/Plan:

- _____
- _____
- _____
- _____
- _____

Nurse Report Sheet

Name:

Code:

Room #:

Allergies:

Isolation:

DX:

PMH:

Neuro:

CV

Resp:

GI/GU:

Skin:

IV'S/Gtt:

Labs:

Notes/Plan:

- _____
- _____
- _____
- _____
- _____

Nurse Report Sheet

Name:

Code:

Room #:

Allergies:

Isolation:

DX:

PMH:

Neuro:

CV

Resp:

GI/GU:

Skin:

IV'S/Gtt:

Labs:

Notes/Plan:
- _____
- _____
- _____
- _____
- _____

🏥 Nurse Report Sheet ∿♡

Name:	Code:	Room #:

Allergies:	Isolation:

DX:

PMH:

Neuro:	CV

Resp:	GI/GU:

Skin:	IV'S/Gtt:

Labs:	Notes/Plan:

Notes/Plan:
- _____
- _____
- _____
- _____
- _____

Nurse Report Sheet

Name:

Code:

Room #:

Allergies:

Isolation:

DX:

PMH:

Neuro:

CV

Resp:

GI/GU:

Skin:

IV'S/Gtt:

Labs:

Notes/Plan:

- _____
- _____
- _____
- _____
- _____

🏥 Nurse Report Sheet ⚕♡

Name:

Code:

Room #:

Allergies:

Isolation:

DX:

PMH:

Neuro:

CV

Resp:

GI/GU:

Skin:

IV'S/Gtt:

Labs:

Notes/Plan:

- _____
- _____
- _____
- _____
- _____